D1662850

MTHFR

Gene Therapy Demystified:

Crack Your Genetic Code to Better Health

Dr. Robin Terranella

Table of Contents

INTRODUCTION

It's simple really, a lot of people are sick and they don't know why or where to start. I know this because these are the people I help every day. The uncertainty stems in part from our limited understanding of health. Despite our limited understanding, we have created a healthcare model that is so common it appears static. That model says, "Fix each single health problem and the whole will be fixed." Like a car that needs a new tire or battery. This is what our medical system is built on, the separation and isolation of individual problems. If you have a thyroid problem it has nothing to do with your digestion and if you have a digestive issue it has nothing to do with your heart. You get the idea.

I went to medical school to study holistic medicine. The medical model of holistic medicine is to understand and treat the whole body as one. The principles were simple and elegant in theory; however, in practice they seemed to rely on the same standard medical system they sought to differentiate from. This model of medicine is so pervasive; it is also quite common in those practicing "holistic medicine". This limited model is at least partially to blame for so much health frustration. Yet, however limited the model is we can use it to expand further if we see it for what it is—limited. Unfortunately, most doctors are not looking to solve your health problems; they are looking to follow an algorithm based on an incomplete model. They are not looking for how all your health problems are connected; instead they are all looking at one particular area that they know a lot about. It takes true curiosity, a willingness to listen and accept that you don't know the answer to truly help. Oftentimes the solutions to health problems are not found where we expect to find them.

Still, knowing this it is easy to fall into the trap of thinking you know the right answer. I have to continually remind myself of this lesson. Yet, even a decision that does not go the way you expect can help you understand the health issue further. This will only work if you are truly invested in problem-solving the health issue. The key is to always ask why.

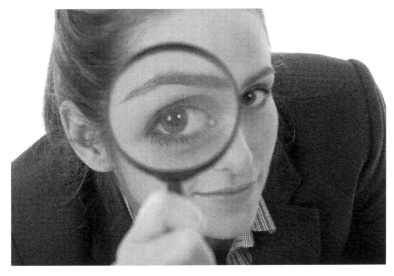

In doing this, I help my patients find the connections between their health symptoms and help them get better. I don't think I do anything particularly unique or genius to help them either. Lots of doctors do the same or similar things. What I use is some old-fashioned careful listening and a burning curiosity. That curiosity is what drives me to find the connections that ultimately help people get better. I hope this book helps you make similar connections.

I have always been curious about how things work in the human body but this curiosity was ignited further when I took a continuing medical education course on genetics and MTHFR by Dr. Ben Lynch. MTHFR is an acronym for methyltetrahydrafolate reductase. It turns out that this one enzyme is connected to many aspects of our health including mood, energy, pain, memory, tissue healing and regeneration, exercise recovery and so much more. Understanding these connections have helped me guide more people to better health. It was the missing formula that promised to unite holistic medicine in the age of modern medicine.

The course was focused on the biochemistry of one enzyme. A

defective MTHFR enzyme causes all sorts of health problems all over the body. My realization (and probably that of others too) was that there are thousands of other enzymes that could cause similar types of problems in other areas of the body. All these variations contribute to health issues and variations in treatment response. This understanding and these connections are the inspiration for this book. I wrote it to help you make similar connections and improve your health.

How to Use This Book

You can think of this book as a foundation for thinking about and understanding your health better. It should give you a clearer three-dimensional complete model to understand your health. As mentioned, western medicine tends to view health through its individual parts and in absolutes. You either have X disease or you don't. This model is very black and white. In my experience many, many people do not fit into these black and white scenarios. That's why I believe this model is unnecessarily limited and incomplete.

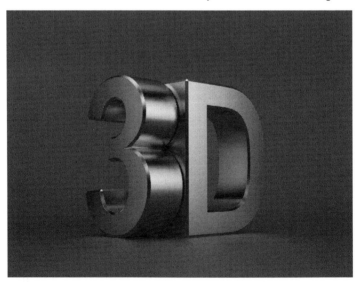

Now, don't get me wrong; modern medicine has solved or improved many health issues and helped many people live longer. The modern medical model has given us a very good outline of human health parameters. For instance, we can now look at many biochemicals in our blood, brain, heart, immune, and digestive system. We can also look at different images, readings, and sounds of our heart, brain, lungs, etc. All this information has helped us define the borders of normal and abnormal. However, what this model has not explored is how and when the normal or abnormal of a given parameter or disease state should be broadened or narrowed based on individual uniqueness. Now that we have the borders defined for much of human health, I suggest it is time to take a more individualistic, refined approach to these borders. When we do this, the black and white will become a more three-dimensional picture. This is where genetics comes in.

Looking at and understanding how genes influence health, biochemistry, physical disease, mental diseases, etc. allows us to see the influence genes have on the parameters of normal and abnormal. We can also more clearly see delineation between nature (genetic) and nurture (environment). While it may not always be crystal clear which has more influence, it is clear that both play a role. Indeed, most health issues are influenced by multiple genes, with each gene being influenced by environmental cues as well. This makes one-size-fits-all protocol based treatments difficult for single gene alterations or disease states.

The benefit of knowing which gene alterations you have is the predictive value. By knowing a gene's function, we can predict how it may affect certain health parameters. An alteration in a single gene can inform us about your health predispositions. I am not saying that just because you have a certain genetic alteration you will have a corresponding lab value or metric that is abnormal; rather, there is a greater chance of having a certain lab value. We have to be aware of the impact from the environment as well.

So having a genetic alteration creates an expected biochemical pattern that is measurable. When we look at your blood levels for certain biochemical, we see how closely they match the expected. Since we know how the enzymes (created by the genes) are supposed to behave, we can track and influence the biochemical pattern so your body and mind operate better. Let's look at an example to make this clearer.

Homocysteine is part of a bigger biochemical process known as methylation (we will discuss methylation in detail below). Homocysteine levels can inform us about your health and treatment progress when you have an MTHFR (methyltetrahydrafolate reductase) genetic alteration. When you have MTHFR enzyme deficiency, we expect you will have high or high normal homocysteine and most people do. Western medicine's normal range for homocysteine is (depending on the lab) 3–12. In many cases a level above 9 and below 5 would signal that something could be off. Above 9 and higher is suggestive of MTHFR gene alteration or a similar under-methylation problem. A lower number could signal over-methylation or similar biochemical pattern. Knowing your genetics and health history allows us to make predictions on certain biochemicals. From this we can gain a better understanding of what is going on when these predictions do and don't match. Do you know what aspects of your biochemistry and labs are off? Are your numbers always "normal"?

If you are feeling confused because no doctor can find out what is wrong with you, the above explanation may make sense to you. Western medicine practitioners make their predictions and reference ranges based on large population studies. In problem solving health issues for the whole of the population, many (maybe you?) have been excluded. You may have been told that you don't quite fit any one problem or disease state. You may have been told that there is nothing you can do or that there is nothing wrong with you. If those comments left you confused, don't be. It is a fact that if you have symptoms, there is something wrong. That health care provider may not know why or have anything to offer but that does not mean you should ignore it or pretend it is normal. Many times you just need a more individualized approach. The tests or treatments that work for most people may not work for you and the answers require digging deeper.

A treatment example that is perhaps pertinent for MTHFR is depression. In most cases people with altered MTHFR genetics do not respond well to pharmaceutical antidepressants. Some feel worse and others don't notice anything from these medications. Very few (with MTHFR) actually see an improvement. There are many other disease and health disordered states that fit a similar pattern. This is due to subtle (or sometimes obvious) genetic variations that don't fit the typical pattern. So what are you to do?

Chances are if you are reading this book, you don't fit into the black and white boxes ascribed by standard medicine. That's ok. While that approach may have fallen short for you, this book will give you a fresh perspective on your unique health situation. I don't pretend it will have all the answers for everyone's health problems. What I have to share with you is an approach to help you better understand your uniqueness. This approach starts with understanding your genetics and the impact environmental factors have on the expression of your genes and health.

This book will specifically be about one of your genes, MTHFR. We will look at the broad reaching effects of the MTHFR gene, the enzymes it affects and the various ways the environment can impact its function. That being said the approach we take to this specific genetic alteration could also be adapted to many other genetic alterations. Before we discuss what to do about having MTHFR, let's first understand a little more about what MTHFR is.

From Genes to Proteins

Before we dive into understanding MTHFR, let's first take a quick detour into a more general topic, your genetic code. To understand what your genetic code is, it helps to understand what DNA is and how it works. Getting this top down understanding will paint a clearer picture of what alterations really mean. This is a bit technical, but hang in there. You don't need to memorize this, just get the gist. Deoxyribonucleic acid, or DNA, is made up of nucleotide base pairs. The available nucleotide base pairs are guanine, cytosine, adenine, and thymine. The "double helix" (see picture) of DNA is created by these base pairs bonding together. Different combinations, lengths, and sequences of these base pairs create your genes. Each gene contains specific sequences of these nucleotide base pairs, which are the instructions for your body to know how to construct proteins.

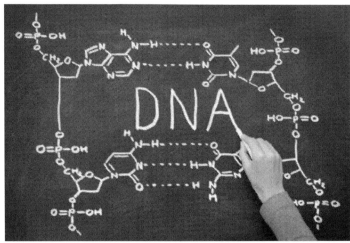

When a nucleotide base in a gene sequence is changed from the "normal", the instructions for the proteins are changed. Because genes can consist of hundreds of nucleotide base pairs, you could have more than one alteration. These alterations can cause a major or minor change or no change in the protein configuration. If the change is common in the population it is a SNP or single nucleotide polymorphism. If it is not very common (less than one percent) it is referred to as a mutation. Both SNPs and mutations are alterations in the gene from the normal (also known as wild type). The MTHFR gene alterations we will be referring to are SNPs.

We can liken a gene to a word and a SNP (or mutation) to a misspelled word. In this analogy the letters are the nucleotide base pairs. When the letters fit together just right, you get a word. When the letters don't fit together, you get something else (gibberish). Depending on which letter is changed you may still be able to make out what the word is. Other times the combination of letters can mean something entirely different or nothing at all. The sequence and configuration of your genes are a lot like this.

The commonality between SNPs and mutations is that both cause a shape change in the resulting protein. A change in shape translates into a change in function. How the new shape interacts with the surrounding molecules is known as spatial configuration.

Spatial configuration of molecules is determined by the charges present in the molecules. Like magnets that attract or oppose one another, the charges present in molecules affect the end shape. When there is a change in the base pairs, the body may use a different amino acid to make the protein. Because each amino acid is charged differently, the shape is altered. A very simplistic way to think about this is to imagine the difference between a strong positive interacting with a strong negative versus two strong positive molecules. This attraction or repulsion creates a dramatic difference in how that protein is shaped. The shape change is how SNPs and mutations change the function of the enzyme.

Instead of just one gene both of our parents each give us a copy of their genes at random. So when the body reads the DNA to make a protein, it is looking at both genes to determine how to make the protein. So if we have an altered nucleotide on one gene and the other is normal, it is referred to as heterozygous. A heterozygous gene alteration is generally going to create a milder protein shape change. On the other hand, when you have two altered genes, one from each parent, you have a homozygous alteration. This is going to cause an alteration in more the proteins (MTHFR enzymes) that are made.

With that compact lesson under our belt, you may be asking, "How can this help me understand my MTHFR alterations?"

That part will come. For now remember that, while your genes are set, your picture of health is only partially determined by your genes. To use the picture analogy, your genetics may create the rough outline but will not determine the whole picture, colors and shades. To understand the full picture we have to understand how genetic and epigenetic influencers work together. It is the combination between genetic and epigenetic influencers that creates your physical, mental, and psychological aspect of what makes you who you are. This is referred to as phenotype. We will discuss epigenetics in more detail below. For now, let's turn our attention to the MTHFR gene itself.

Step 1:
Determine Severity

What Is MTHFR?

All enzymes are proteins that allow biochemical reactions to occur with greater ease. They assist our bodies in converting and changing molecules in our bodies. The alterations in genetics we are concerned with affect these enzymes. The MTHFR enzyme converts inactive folate like folic acid into active folate or 5-MTHF. An alteration in the genes causes decreased 5-MTHF levels. Without going into all the numerous case scenarios that could present as a result of having MTHFR alteration, I want you to have enough information to understand how I approach the treatment. If you found out that you had an altered MTHFR enzyme, the obvious question that would come to mind would be, "How much methylfolate, or 5-MTHF, do I need to take?" There are so many varying opinions and dosages. How do you know how much is right for your body? This is exactly what we are going to discuss together.

Before we can determine how much methylfolate you do or do not need to take, we need to know how severe your SNPs is. If you already know, bear with me as this is important. Before we discuss severity I want you to understand what it is that this gene is actually doing in our body.

The MTHFR gene is one of the most highly studied genes in humans. So we actually know quite a bit about what happens when there are alterations. The MTHFR gene is the code for the MTHFR enzyme. The enzyme allows your body convert inactive folate (like folic acid) to an active folate (L-methylfolate). Seems simple enough on the surface and it is when we look at this reaction in isolation. However, the way your body uses methyfolate is much more dynamic and dimensional. You see methylfolate is a very bioactive substance. When present, it reacts with many other molecules and causes many different biochemical reactions. The main biochemical pathway that methylfolate is connected to is called methylation.

The process of methylation is really passing one molecule (a methyl group) along to another. When this happens, it changes the effect and activity level of the molecule being methylated. A methyl group is a carbon with three hydrogens attached to it. In the process involving metylfoalte, homocysteine is converted into methionine and then SAMe (S-adenosylmethionine) via this process. SAMe is the prize product of methylation and does the bulk of methyl group donating. I know this may be a bit confusing but think of methylation like passing the baton. Once the next molecule takes the baton (from SAMe) a lot of other reactions are permitted to take place.

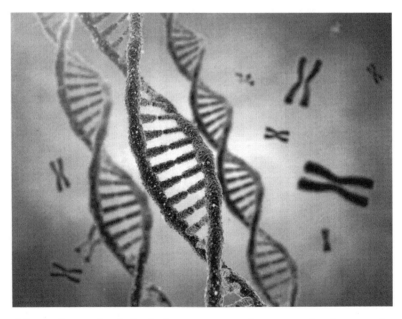

Many key physiological processes in your body require a methylation step. For instance, choline is produced through the methylation process. This important molecule allows us to think clearly via acetylcholine and allows us to have proper cell membrane structure and cell signaling via phosphatidylcholine. Phosphatidylcholine is also an important protective component of many mucus membranes and is needed for myelin sheath formation. Through its relation to the above, choline, and by default, MTHFR, is implicated in Alzheimer's Disease (acetylcholine), Multiple Sclerosis (myelin sheath), chronic nutrient deficiencies (via poor cell membranes), and inflammation in mucus membrane dependent on mucus production. When there is a deficiency in methylfolate, there is likely a deficiency in phosphatidylcholine too, since you need one to get the other.

So, just like that, methylation has connections to many chronic health issues. A simple search on your favorite search engine will show that there are many correlations between MTHFR and the above mentioned chronic health issues. However, only about 35% of the methylation process in your body is used to make phosphatidyle choline. What else does methylation do? Another 35% of methylation goes to making creatine.

Yes creatine the stuff body builders take. Ceatine plays a very active role in energy production throughout your body. It is particularly needed in those tissues with higher energy demands like the muscles and brain. The role of creatine is to recycle energy molecules from ADP (adenosine diphosphate) to ATP (adenosine triphosphate) by adding a phosphate. This gives the body an alternative route for making energy and acts as a buffer for energy reserves. Creatine is produced and used by the body regularly. It is particularly useful when energy demands are higher like when exercising. The enzyme that produces creatine is GAMT (guanidinoacetate methyltransferase). This enzyme also needs SAMe to make creatine. Deficiencies in this enzyme (GAMT) cause cognitive, behavioral, neurological, and musculoskeletal issues [1]. Because of GAMT's need for SAMe, a deficiency in methylfolate will have a similar effect.

Now, with 70% of methylation accounted for what else does methylation do? The remaining 30% is used for:

- Removal of toxins from your body/detox (including histamine)
- Artery responsiveness (nitric oxide production)
- Responding to infections
- DNA repair
- Turning DNA on and off
- and more

So this is the purpose of methylation and in the process of methylation MTHFR helps in the formation of SAMe. SAMe does the heavy lifting (or baton passing) of methyl donation and alterations in the MTHFR enzyme interrupt the production of SAMe. The severity of your MTHFR gene SNPs will determine how slowed the methylation process will be. There are two main MTHFR SNPs on the MTHFR gene. When these SNPs are present they do impact the enzyme's function. However, this enzyme is not the only one that can affect methylation. There are several other enzymes in the process of methylation that can also effect the overall cycle. Some of these will be discussed below. Before we get too far into this, I think it is worthwhile for you to take an inventory of what exactly your health problems are.

This is exactly what I do with my patients in the office before I even consider giving advice on what to do about MTHFR. This is such an overlooked part of the process. For starters, you have to know where you are at now to fully appreciate any changes that may take place as a result of treating your MTHFR. You may say, "Well, I feel bad, isn't that enough?" No, it's too vague and will lead to a vague notion of how treating your MTHFR defect is helping. Possibly even worse is that the side effect that could happen from taking methylfolate could go unnoticed.

It is also important since there are many things that MTHFR treatment will not help or should be treated separately before treating MTHFR. In fact, while I have helped a lot of people with MTHFR gene defects, I don't think of myself as treating MTHFR. I treat the person and all aspects of their health. My approach to this will be discussed below. First, take some time to answer the questions below. This will start to create an honest depiction of your current health state. These are some, but not all, of the questions I typically use.

Health Evaluation

General Symptoms

Make a list of symptoms you think you need help with and rate their severity from 1 to 10.

Those questions that have higher severity should be given more priority. Cross reference these symptoms with the common MTHFR symptoms and associated health conditions listed below (and other sources). See if your most severe symptoms correlate with the most common MTHFR symptoms.

Common MTHFR Symptoms

- *Fatigue*
- *Depression*
- *Anxiety*
- *Neuropathy*
- *Other Nerve problems*
- *Headaches and Migraines*
- *High Blood Pressure*

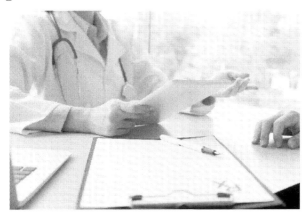

Common Associated Health Conditions

- *Multiple Sclerosis*
- *Fibromyalgia*
- *Infertility (male and female)*
- *Chemical Sensitivity*
- *Tongue Tie*
- *Parkinson's*
- *Spina Bifida*
- *Schizophrenia*
- *IBS*
- *Allergies*
- *Asthma*
- *Eczema*
- *Cancer (multiple)*
- *Blood Clots*
- *Addiction*
- *Autism*
- *Down Syndrome*
- *Epilepsy*
- *Type 1 Diabetes*
- *Cardiovascular Disease*

List created from my clinical background and enhanced with the help of <u>Dr. Lynch.</u>[2]

If you have other symptoms not related to MTHFR, consider treating those first or separately. Remember MTHFR is connected to a lot of biochemical pathways so there is a chance this symptom will get better from improving your MTHFR and methylation.

Do you have trouble with weight loss or gain?

This may not be related to MTHFR unless you have digestive problems. Outside of digestion consider getting screened for hormonal issues, which can cause weight gain or loss. This is a starting place; many things can cause weight gain or loss.

Digestion

- Do you have any gas, bloating or abdominal pain?

Abdominal pain will be obvious but gas and bloating you may be used to. Take a real honest look at this. If you are feeling this way often, you may not be digesting your food well or you may have a microbial imbalance. More on this below.

- Do you have acid reflux, take medications for acid reflux or any medications for your digestion?

- Do you have at least one bowel movement daily?

If not, you should address this depending on how bad it is. There are several reasons for constipation.

- Do you have to avoid a lot of different foods?

When people have multiple food sensitivities it suggests you may have pathogenic microbe, SIBO, histamine intolerance or some other digestive problem. This is especially the case when the sensitivities get worse over time.

- When you go off this more restricted diet do your bowel movements change a lot?

- Do you feel like you can eat whatever you want?

If that is the case, good for you. Still I recommend looking more closely at the relationship between the foods you eat and some of the questions above.

Optimal digestion is key for optimal health. If you are going to start taking methylfolate you might as well absorb it.

Energy

- How is your energy (scale 1–10)?

- Do you have brain fog?

- How is your exercise recovery compared to your younger self or peers?

If you have low energy, brain fog and poor exercise recovery, all these could be related to MTHFR.

Do you have trouble sleeping or want to sleep all the time?

Poor sleep could be caused by or connected to MTHFR. However, more often methylfolate can make sleep worse. Be careful if you already have sleep issues.

Neurological

- Do you have numbness and tingling in any part of your body?

- Do you have pain that is neurological?

- Do you have headaches?

All these could be related to MTHFR.

Psychological

- How is your mood?

- Have you been diagnosed with depression, anxiety or Bipolar disorder?

- Do you find it difficult to be happy and upbeat?

- Do you worry about things constantly?

If you have these types of symptoms or been diagnosed it could be related to your MTHFR gene.

Based on the above information you should now have a better overall idea of what health problems need to be addressed. In the sections that follow I will discuss specifics on how severe your particular MTHFR SNP might be and how this relates to your symptoms and approach to treatment. We will also be discussing some of the other health issues that may have come up in the quiz.

SNP Severity

So now that you have an idea of why the MTHFR gene is important, let's look at the different levels of gene alteration that the SNPs cause. The MTHFR gene is highly susceptible to alteration by polymorphic areas in the gene. Most research suggests that there are two main SNPs that have a significant impact MTHFR enzyme. There likely are others but they are either very rare (and potentially more problematic) or don't really affect the end function of the MTHFR enzyme much. The two SNPs that we know are problematic are positioned at C677T and A1298C. Because all humans have two copies of every gene, you could have a few different combinations of these SNPs at these places on the MTHFR gene.

The general idea is that you take on one copy from your mom and one copy from your dad. If Mom and Dad have no SNPs in their genes then you will not have any either. If either parent has two copies of one of the SNPs, then you will end up with at least one SNP on the MTHFR gene from that one parent.

Of the two SNPs, the one that alters the MTHFR enzyme the most is C677T. When you have two copies of this SNP, <u>your MTHFR enzyme will be reduced by approximately 70%</u>.[3] This means the enzyme works at 70% less efficiency than it would in someone with the normal variations. Some research suggests it is reduced by more than 70% but these are both estimates. In any case, the reduced enzyme activity leads to reduced methylfolate for your body to use. As a result there is a reduction in all the processes noted above. The A1298C MTHFR SNP also reduces the enzyme activity (see below for specifics).

How relevant are these SNPs and do they really affect enough people to matter? The answer is it depends. I have treated people with MTHFR SNPs and it completely changed their life. I have also seen people with major SNPs who did not even know they had a health issue. Once we treated it, however, they did feel better. It is estimated that some form of an MTHFR SNP affects up to 50% of the population. Below are some of the specific combinations and their estimated affect on the enzyme function.

C677T
One copy - 30% decline
Two copies - 70% decline

A1298C
One copy – 10–15% decline
Two copies – 40–50% decline

Compound Heterozygous
One copy of each - 60% decline

Now that you have an idea how altered your MTHFR enzyme is, what do you do about it? The SNPs you have allow us to predict how likely you are to have a methylation problem but there are many ways this can manifest. To go back to the picture analogy from earlier, your MTHFR gene might determine the color but the environmental epigenetic factors decide the shades of color in the picture.

Step 2:
Epigenetics and Overall Health

Epigenetics refers to changes that occur on our chromosome (where the genes are seated) that do not change the underlying genes but do change the gene activity. Classically this terminology refers to chromosomal modification that would only be passed on to offspring. Here we are using the term epigenetics more loosely. We are using it to refer to environmental triggers that can alter our genes throughout our lifespan and those that are hereditable. One interesting fact often attributed to epigenetic factors is the relationship between the number of proteins versus the number of genes coding for proteins. Indeed, the number of proteins that make up our human bodies is somewhere around 70,000. Yet the number of genes found to code for proteins is a mere 20,000. That is a big difference. If our human characteristics were simply determined by the variations in the 20,000 genes then those other 50,000 proteins would not matter much. But we know this is not true. In fact, what has been shown is that the body takes cues from the environment. These cues turn on and off promoter and inhibitor areas on our genes. The intersection of environment with genetics is critical because this interaction creates all the shades, structure, and color of you as a person and your health. To fully optimize your health you have to be able to manipulate the environment inside as a whole. We will come back to the importance and perspectives of single genes after visiting some basic internal environmental manipulation.

What do I mean by environment?

Your body's internal environment is made up of the chemicals present to form your biochemistry. It is the blood, the cells, metabolites, macronutrients, micronutrients and everything in between. Of course, we don't have to know and understand all these biochemicals to manipulate your internal environment and optimize your health. Here we will focus on the necessary steps that are essential for optimal methylation and MTHFR gene function.

If you don't take these steps first, this lack of attention will limit your health improvements. These are so important that in some cases I would say it doesn't even make sense to look at your genetics until these are addressed. That is not to say MTHFR is not important but more that the importance is drowned out by the bigger health issues caused by a poor internal environment. As such, when you begin to support your genetic imbalances, it will take a lot more effort. And in the end, and after a lot of effort, you may not notice a thing. With this in mind we will discuss the 5 key areas to optimize (to the extent possible) and why they are important.

Step 3:
Prepping for Methylfolate

The process of prepping for methylfolate consumption is essentially creating the most optimal environment for the MTHFR enzyme (and all enzymes) to thrive in. The five areas are:

1. The food you eat

2. The absorption of the food

3. Toxin elimination

4. Immune system activity

5. Inflammation

1. Nutrition and the Food You Eat

At the heart of genetics is biochemistry and at the heart of biochemistry are enzymes. Enzymes are what allow the thousands of different biochemical structures floating around in your body to exist. The starting material for these enzymes is the food you eat.

So nutrition is literally the fuel that keeps your body going. It is also how you create energy and rebuild damaged areas in your body. The food you eat can do much more than this though. For instance, eating too much of the wrong foods can cause inflammatory, immune, digestive, endocrine and other health issues. Equally problematic is eating too little of the right foods, causing tissue wasting, impaired neurological, immune, endocrine, and other organ and tissue dysfunction. Of course, eating too much overall is not good either.

Too much bad, too much in general and too little in general will not specifically impact the MTHFR enzyme (although some specific nutritional things do and will be discussed), but they will affect your health. When you start treating MTHFR, if you don't have a good foundation for your health, you won't notice much difference or you may feel worse.

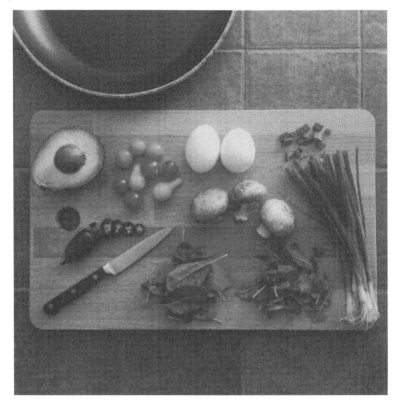

Let's look at **eating too much of the wrong or bad food** first. What constitutes wrong food? Generally this refers to foods that make you feel bad or have specific detrimental health effects. The main thing that eating the wrong food does is trigger or promote inflammation. How do you know which foods are triggering inflammation?

Inflammation occurs for various reasons and has many sources. One common source is food. Some foods can trigger inflammation because of how the food interacts with the immune system in close proximity to the digestive tract. A detailed discussion of this can be found in the "absorption of food" section below.

On a more macro level, some foods are greater promoters of

inflammation. The promotion of inflammation has more to do with the omega 3 - omega 6 fatty acid ratios in your overall diet. When you have an excess of omega 6, it leads to more inflammation. It works like this. The cells of your body are made up of fats and they are constantly colliding with toxins both from the environment and those created by the body. When this collision occurs, the fatty part of the cell membrane is damaged and a piece is broken off. This broken off portion acts as a signal; the signal is recognized by the immune system. These signals can either be pro-inflammation molecules or anti-inflammation molecules. When the broken piece of fatty acid comes from an omega 6 fat, pro-inflammation signals are produced. When the broken piece of fat comes from an omega 3 fatty acid, anti-inflammation signals are produced. The key thing to remember is excess omega 6 to omega 3. Our bodies do need both to function but too much omega 6 leads to excess inflammation.

So what is excess omega 6? You should have a 1:3–1:6 ratio of omega 3 to omega 6. On average humans consume too much omega 6 and not enough omega 3, about a 1:12 ratio. A common misconception is all omegas are good for you. This is true relative to saturated and hydrogenated fats, but in the vast majority of cases this does not mean you should supplement with omega 6. If you are supplementing with omega fats make it omega 3s. How do you know if you need these at all? The typical rule of thumb is if you are eating fish (wild caught, cold water) more than twice per week you probably don't need more (unless otherwise directed by a healthcare provider). Otherwise a supplement may be needed. You can also test your omega 3/6 ratio via a blood test to find out.

Toxins like heavy metals, pesticides, insecticides, and other chemicals in your food can also be a source of inflammation as they are the initial start to the cell membrane damage. While all sources of inflammation are very important, there are some finer details of this topic that are beyond the scope of this book. We will discuss toxins in more detail below.

Macronutrients

So what about **not eating enough of the good foods**? By "good foods" I mean the macronutrients (protein, fats, and carbs) and micronutrients (vitamins, minerals, etc.) required to have sufficient (and optimal) health.

Macronutrients are the carbohydrates, fats and proteins that make up the food we eat. Your body needs enough protein for a normal immune system, hormonal system, brain function, muscle recovery, etc. Outside of water the majority of your body is made up of protein.

If we look a little closer the proteins we eat are really made up of amino acids. So it is the amino acids that are really needed, not so much protein. Some of these amino acids the body can manufacture and some it cannot. The ones that it cannot manufacture are called essential amino acids. They are histidine, isoleucine, leucine, lysine, methionine, phenylalanine, threonine, tryptophan, and valine. So how much protein (amino acids) do you need? About 1/2 of your body weight in grams of protein. This is a rough figure and can change based on your goals, exercise, specific health issues.

Fats are in some ways the forgotten macronutrient in the sense that they have been mainly pushed aside for the last 20 to 40 yrs. Despite their lack of popularity in the past, your body will not run very well without enough fat in your diet. Your body needs fats to make hormones, cell membranes, and other crucial aspects of your health. The minimum fat necessary is about 10% of your total calories but a larger amount up to 70% can also be considered healthy if you are following a ketogenic eating plan, for instance.

Small amounts of carbohydrates are also needed, specifically for your brain and kidneys to survive, but your body can also manufacture small amounts of these from protein. Generally speaking, you need to have at least 15–20% of your overall macronutrients from carbohydrates. Most people consume far too many carbohydrates

(50% or more) leading to insulin resistance, diabetes, weight gain, heart disease, hypoglycemia, and many other health ailments. A feeling of low blood sugar (carbs) or hypoglycemia can be triggered shortly after (30 to 90 minutes) consuming large amounts of sugar or carbohydrate. This feeling is caused by a cortisol or epinephrine spike leading to an anxiety or stress response, often followed by a crash in energy. This zigzag in energy and mood is common in people consuming high carbohydrate diets. If you have anxiety or mood swings, look at stabilizing your blood sugar as a way to help control this. It should be noted that most non-root vegetable sources of carbohydrates (like spinach and lettuce) should not be limited in this context.

Micronutrients

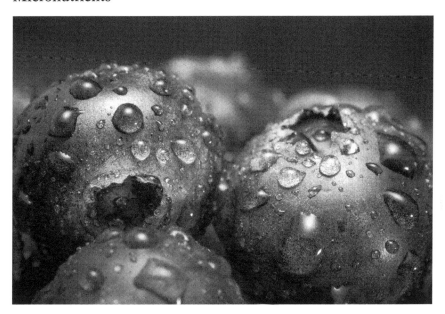

On the micronutrients side of nutrition, vitamins, minerals, and other nutrients are needed to keep the processes of the body working as they should. I think of these like the grease that keeps the gears in the machine running. The vitamins and minerals are co-factors for many key enzymatic processes to work. That is why they are so important and why adding specific ones can be so helpful. In fact, MTHFR is one of these enzymes. It makes methylfolate and this methylfolate provides the grease for another enzyme, methionine synthase (MTR), to work. So where do these mysterious micronutrients and vitamins come from? You guessed it, mainly fruits and vegetables but animal products too.

If you have MTHFR and are not sure how much methylfolate to take (I will explain this in detail below) a great place to start is with dark, leafy greens (uncooked). You can get active folate (methylfolate) directly from these and this is one of the safest ways to give you small but consistent doses. These will also give you many other vitamins and minerals. Try to eat some dark, leafy greens like salad once daily. We will discuss more diet considerations for MTHFR below in Section 4.

Now that we have discussed the importance of all those nutrients what do you think happens when your digestion is compromised and you cannot absorb those nutrients? (See the next section for the answer.)

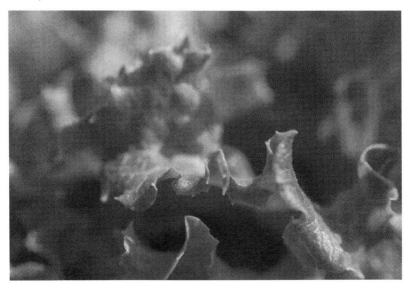

Action Step:

1. Consider supplementing with Omega 3 fatty acids based on the information provided.

2. Try to remove other toxins from your diet. Look up The Dirty Dozen.

3. Evaluate your macronutrient balance and ask yourself how much protein, fat and carbohydrates are in my diet.

4. Eat salad or dark, leafy greens 5–7 days per week.

2. Digestion

A healthy digestive tract is important for many reasons but the most basic one has to do with absorption of nutrients. Your digestion also primes your immune system and as a result can contribute to many health problems. Of course, your body's ability to break down the food you eat and turn it into energy is largely attributed to the digestive tract. The transformation of food into usable energy requires a coordinated effort across many different systems. For instance, your stomach needs to have enough acids, your small intestine needs enough enzymes, the digestive muscles need to be coordinated and responsive, endocrine hormones signaling, and just the right amount of nervous system input. When these digestive functions are insufficient, uncoordinated, and generally not working right, you end up with less extraction of the nutrients from your food. So even if you are eating great you may not be getting much from it.

You can think of the extraction of nutrients from your food like a vacuum sucking the nutrients out. The power of the vacuum is dependent on the villi and microvilli in the small intestine. These are the finger-like and hair-like projections that allow for such small particles to get into the body. Inflammatory foods, toxins, infections, and food sensitivities can damage this delicate tissue, leading to impaired absorption and many other problems. Because the immune system is in such close proximity to the intestine (wrapped around them) the impact of food is critical.

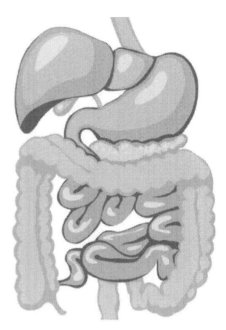

When you consume foods your immune system sees as a threat, it gets primed for inflammation. Just like a potential microbial threat, a food threat will trigger an immune response and attack. This leads to local inflammation and damage to the mucosa (villi and microvilli). These signals can also be transmitted (in a weaker sense) to the entire body. This can also leave you and your immune system more susceptible to colds, flu, autoimmune reactions and infections in general.

Also, if you currently have, or in the past had, damage to the digestive tract (particularly the small intestines) and you have an MTHFR defect you may need additional support to rebuild the villi and microvilli noted above. Any rapidly dividing cell like hair, skin, and digestive cells requires a lot of DNA and as such is highly methylation dependent. Because MTHFR is critical for methylation this could cause a problem for nutrient absorption. In some cases I will give methylfolate as an intramuscular shot along with B12 and other nutrients depending on how severe the absorption issues are.

So what should you do and what does this have to do with MTHFR? The first thing is to work on improving your digestion and find out if you have digestive issues (a full discussion on this topic is outside the scope of this book). But don't make the mistake of overlooking a potential problem and/or thinking that since no one has diagnosed a digestive issue you don't have one. If you do have digestive issues, no matter how insignificant they seem, I recommend fixing these before you start taking methylfolate. This is bolded for a reason, it's important. If you don't fix your digestive issues more than likely the folate will make you sick (nausea, headaches, rash) or will not work very well for you. When someone comes to me and says they tried methylfolate and they did not get any better or it made them worse, I always look to the digestive tract as the culprit.

Action Step

1. Take a mental inventory of your digestive system symptoms. Do you have issues like gas, bloating, pain, constipation, diarrhea, loose stools or inconsistent stools?

2. Check out the Bristol Stool chart to compare your stools with what is considered normal. Many times what you assume is normal may not be, so be sure to find out.

3. Learn more about or get tested for food sensitivities and triggers and remove all of these from your diet.

4. For more details see a doctor that can evaluate your digestion or check out my online course Digestive Reset.[4]

3. Detoxification

A critical part of optimal health revolves around your body's efficient and effective removal of the toxins it encounters. Your body inherently generates molecules that it then has to eliminate and detoxify from every day. This occurs constantly and is part of the normal biochemical processes. Typically these molecules are relatively easy for our bodies to eliminate because they are congruent with our biochemistry.

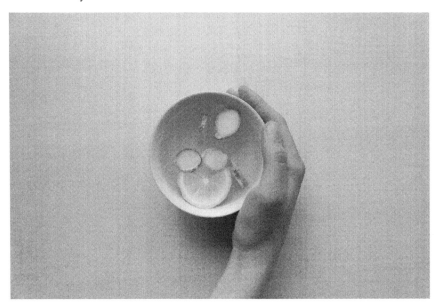

However, our environment is steadily increasing it's accumulation of toxic man-made molecules from multiple industries. The vegetables and fruits you eat are only one source. The air you breathe, the water you drink and clean with, the furniture you sit on, clothes you wear, items you eat off of, etc., are all sources of toxins. So much of what we encounter on a daily basis is saturated with these foreign chemicals and our bodies have to get rid of them.

If you are unable to eliminate these toxins, they are left to float in the bloodstream and can get deposited in our fat and other tissues where they cause cell damage and inflammation. These toxins can disrupt many of the processes in our body leading to impaired endocrine function, decreased immunity, and inflammation. The reason why some people have problems with this and others don't comes down to two things—your past and current exposures and your unique genetics.

There are multiple routes by which all toxins can exit the body but usually there is one preferred route for each toxin. Each route is driven by different enzymes, each of which can have genetic alteration that can speed up or slow down its efficiency. Where genetic impairment and exposures overlap is when people can develop health problems. You can think about detoxification like a highway network. The cars are the toxins and the roads are the enzymes that help the body remove the toxins. When one road gets filled up, the cars have to choose a different route. This can then lead to additional roads being congested. The more roads that are congested the more the cars (toxins) cause problems with cellular function.

Many pesticides and insecticides work by targeting the DNA of the organism. These same toxins can interrupt your DNA replication, leading to mutations or alteration in protein enzyme function. Heavy metals like lead and mercury negatively affect the body in many ways too. One pertinent way is through interruption of enzyme function. For instance, both lead and mercury down-regulate methione synthase[5] (MTR), the same enzyme methylfolate helps to work. The chemical found in many plastics, BPA, interrupts methyltransferase enzymes needed for cell membrane production (PEMT), neurotransmitter production (BH4), creatine production (GAMT) and others.

Many people who have MTHFR mutations are very sensitive to perfumes, smells and other environmental toxins. This is a symptom of overflowing and clogged detoxification pathways. Because of this you should try to create an optimal environment for your body's enzymes to do their job. To do this stay away from and helping to promote the elimination of toxins.

Action Step

1. Consider doing a short (24 hr.) focused detox once weekly or once monthly that includes all organic foods, no animal products, sauna (or some form of increased sweating), increased fiber intake (go slow but gradually increase), herbs (like milk thistle) and nutrients to enhance the elimination of toxins.

2. Look at your exposure to toxins in your daily life and find ways to reduce the sources of the toxins. Focus on your home or bedroom since you spend most time there. Some ideas include reducing smells from cleaning, clothes, and perfumes. You can also reduce your use of non-stick pans for cooking. Avoid eating or drinking from plastics. Reduce the use of pesticides and insecticides near and in your home. Environmental Working Group at EWG.org[6] is a good resource for this.
Also look at The Dirty Dozen and The Clean 15 to find ways to reduce your consumption of these as well.

4. Immune System and Infections

Fatigue is a common symptom associated with MTHFR and many people with Chronic Fatigue Syndrome have problems with methylation. However, those methylation issues are not always coming from a genetic source (like MTHFR). Sometimes they have an infectious origin.

When I am working with a patient, there are specific symptoms that lead me to believe their fatigue is from an infectious source. The main one is mild flu-like symptoms (body aches and joint aches) that come and go. Ot Fatigue that comes and goes. Many times people think they keep getting sick but really it is the microbe changing from an active to dormant state. This may seem a little odd, so let me explain this in a little more detail.

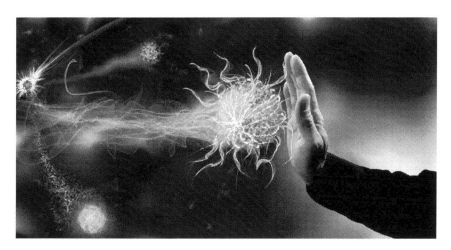

Cold and flu symptoms are a normal part of human existence. The symptoms are caused by the immune system's response to the bug. In some cases people cannot get rid of viruses and bacteria efficiently and they linger in the body at low levels for months and even years. Most of the time, the microbes oscillate between dormant and active stages. During the active flare-ups you feel like you might have the flu, fatigue, and joint aches. These flares could last a few hours to a few days or even longer.

A common, better known example of this is with the Herpes Zoster virus also known as shingles. Shingles is simply a reactivation of the common chickenpox virus.

The same scenario happens with Epstein Bar virus (and others). This virus is the cause of a condition known as mononucleosis and is highly implicated as a factor in causing Chronic Fatigue Syndrome. As noted, many people with Chronic Fatigue Syndrome go through periods of "flare-ups" and this is thought to occur when the virus is reactivated. In normal circumstances the virus lives in the nerve roots but is suppressed by the immune system. Those with Chronic Fatigue Syndrome cannot keep the virus suppressed. It should be noted that not all people with the syndrome have a chronic viral or other infection as the cause.

So why does one person have a flare-up of these viruses and the next person does not? One reason is based on genetic susceptibility. There are a few major and some minor genetic problems that can affect the immune system in this way. Immunoglobulins are like GPS tracking devices that the immune system creates to identify and isolate pathogens (viruses, bacteria, etc). The white blood cells make these after exposure to pathogens. The immunoglobulins are used in the body when we are exposed to the same pathogen in the future. This allows the immune system to react to it faster. There are different types of immunoglobulins for different areas of the body and for different types of pathogens. The four different types are IgA, IgG, IgM, and IgE. All four can have genetic problems that occur with them both in how the body produces them and how they function once they are made.

For instance, with an immunoglobulin deficiency of IgG or IgA, your body will have more trouble getting rid of the viruses, bacteria or other microbes. The microbes themselves and the inflammation they create impair many enzymes from working properly, including the ones in the methylation cycle. It is not hard to see that someone with immunoglobulin deficiency will have trouble with chronic infections. However, chronic infections can and do occur in people with a "normal" immune system as well.

Action Step

1. How is your immune system working? How often have you been "sick" in the last 12–18 months? Do you have chronic allergies, hives or skin reactions?

2. If so, take a deep look at your immune system. Specifically focus on the relationship of your digestive system to these symptoms. When you have digestive problems do you feel sicker and vice versa? Follow the steps in the digestive section to try to improve those problems. Remember your digestive tract primes your immune system.

3. Consider being tested for immunoglobulin levels and for chronic infections like EBV, CMV, HHSV-6, and others. There is also a functional test for immune system by Spectra Cell Labs that can help you understand how your white blood cells respond to pathogens.

5. Inflammation

Inflammation is really at the center of every health issue humans face. All of the above problems—toxins, infections, digestion, poor absorption of nutrients—are problematic because they cause, worsen or lead to inflammation. Inflammation comes from your immune system, which works best when there is good digestion.

Action Step

1. Ensure you are getting proper amounts of omega 3 fatty acids and consider having a test done to see what your ratio is.
2. Ensure your digestive tract is optimized; consider having a further evaluation done if there is uncertainty.
3. Follow steps to toxin elimination and consider having GGT tested on a standard test and heavy metals urine provocation test.
4. Inflammation in the blood can be checked and approximated with tests like CRP, hsCRP, ESR, elevated antibody levels, albumin/globulin ratio, elevated liver enzyme; however, just because they are negative or normal does not mean you don't have inflammation. If they are elevated then you know you have inflammation.
5. If these are high, try to get them down before moving on to step 4.

Step 4:
Dosing

How Much Methylfolate Should I Take?

The dose of folate you need is always going to depend on your unique health and genetic situation. To start with, remember that MTHFR is only one of about twenty thousand genes in your body. In some cases you could be made worse by taking folate, so be careful. When you correct one genetic defect, you may create other unforeseen side effects, which I will discuss below.

When I am trying to determine the dose of methylfolate for someone to take, I keep the following things in mind:

- The Person's Symptoms

- Their Medical History

- Their Current Diet and Lifestyle

- Their Specific MTHFR Genes

- Other Known (or presumptive) Genetic Alterations

Your Symptoms

Not everyone who has an MTHFR mutation needs to take methylfolate every day or at all. This is true even if you have a more severe alteration like the C677T described above. The symptoms that make me think you should be taking methylfolate are fatigue, depression, brain fog, anxiety, numbness or neuropathy of any kind. If you don't have these but you do have a moderate to severe mutation, you may consider taking a dose of methylfolate periodically (a few times per week). During times when you are under more stress you may also need more. Just be careful as taking too much could lead to feeling more pressure and anxiety. This may sound contradictory, but the reasons for this will be described in the section below.

If you do have these symptoms, the methylfolate will likely help you, but pay attention to the other influencers on the dose of methylfolate.

Medical History

In step 3 we described the reasons why having a good digestive and immune system are important, the main one being that when they are not good, your body has more inflammation, disrupting the activity of many of the enzymes (especially in the methylation cycle). Therefore, if you have a mild version of MTHFR but it seems like you have all the symptoms of MTHFR mutation, you may be tempted to take more methylfolate. If it helps, great; but if it does not, revisit these steps as a potential source of your frustration.

Another (and likely more successful) option is to treat and resolve those other (digestive, toxic, immune) issues first. This is what I recommend, and when you do this, you are likely to have better results when you do take the methylfolate. Similarly, if you have a moderate to severe MTHFR alteration but are not improving or possibly getting worse (from taking methylfolate) consider looking more closely at some of these other factors.

Current Diet and Lifestyle

The specific diet recommendations for those with MTHFR are to avoid folic acid and to try to get folate from dark, leafy greens. Since folic acid is fortified in most grains (rice, wheat, and corn meal) reducing grain consumption will typically have a big impact. Keep in mind that reducing grains can reduce the amount of other B vitamins in your diet like B6. Cutting back on grains can also have health benefits aside from their effect on methylation. Folic acid is also found in many multivitamins but you can get one with methylfolate instead.

Note that folic acid is also used as filler in many medications, especially if they are compounded.

The reason folic acid is bad for people with MTHFR mutation is because methylfolate has to be transported through the body on a carrier protein. The same carrier protein that transports methylfolate also carries folic acid. So if you are consuming folic acid, all the carriers are bound with folic acid and cannot transport your methylfolate. Therefore, the dose of methylfolate you consume is not going to do much for your body because it is relatively small compared to the folic acid. So before consuming methylfolate start by reducing or eliminating grains.

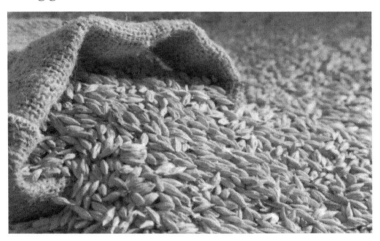

In addition, some people have genetic alterations in this carrier protein itself (SLC19a1), making it more difficult to transport all folates. When this is present, reducing folic acid in your diet is even more critical.

Another dietary consideration is your consumption of alcohol and/or caffeine. Both increase your body's demand for methylfolate and other B vitamins. So if you are consuming alcohol you may need more methylfolate than we would otherwise think. Remember, though, alcohol and other toxins can lead to oxidative stress and inflammation.

Inflammation disrupts how the enzymes in methylation work. So don't think you can simply continue to consume alcohol and just take more methylfolate. You have to remove the toxins, too, and be sure to eat things that neutralize the oxidative stress like the antioxidants found in fruits and veggies. That's why you can never go wrong by getting extra folate from your diet. Folate comes from dark, leafy greens like kale, spinach, chard, and mixed greens, and these also have antioxidants. Remember you cannot out supplement a poor diet.

See this reference chart[7] for other medications to avoid when possible. This is not me telling you to stop these medications but to consider other options (with your doctor) when you have an MTHFR mutation.

Your Specific MTHFR Alteration and Dosing Considerations

In light of everything written above you may want a general idea of how much folate you should take. These are general guidelines from my experience with patients. Ultimately, the decision of how much to take will be up to you, your treatment team, and your response. Periodic testing of homocysteine (and other methylation cycle markers like SAM/SAH) can help you better understand what your optimal dose is. However, homocysteine alone will not tell you what dose you should be taking. All the information needs to be put into context together.

C677T

One copy - 30% decline

- 800–4,000 mcg per day

Two copies - 70% decline

- 5,000–15,000 mcg per day

A1298C

One copy – 10–15% decline

- no extra folate needed.

Two copies – 40–50% decline

2000–4000 mcg per day

Compound Heterozygous

One copy of each - 60% decline

- 5,000–15,000 mcg per day

Also please note that these are very generalized dosing ideas. Sometimes you have to start much lower and work up. Once you start feeling better you may need to reduce the dose a bit. Many people feel worse if they maintain higher dosing levels for long periods. Then you may find that you have to increase the dose beyond what it originally was. This is your body finding new ways to make use of the methylfolate. The timing on when to increase and decrease cannot be predicted. When I am working with someone to determine this, I base it on clinical insight (how the person responds to specific questions). You should have a good idea based on the information provided here and below.

Other variables that may change the dose you take can be the stressors in your life and other genetic factors discussed below. So use this referencing dosing as a general and not a static guide.

Other Genetic Alterations

Let's face it, genetics can be confusing. Since most people get interested in genetics though the lens of MTHFR, I am going to lay out other genetic alternation in relation to MTHFR. Some of the genetic alterations that can change the amount of methylfolate I recommend include:

- COMT - decrease

- MAOA and MAOB - decrease

- SOD/CAT- decrease

- SUOX - decrease

- CBS (C699T) - decrease

- MTR- increase

- MTRR- increase

- GAMT - increase

- PEMT - increase

- BHMT- increase

- FOL1 - increase

Notice how they would affect the dosing of your methylfolate with "increased" or "decreased" next to it. Let's look at a few of these specifically.

Decrease

The COMT (catechol-o-methyl transferase) enzyme works to help the body break down catecholamine neurotransmitters like dopamine and epinephrine (as well as estrogens and xenoestrogens). The most relevant COMT SNP is the V158M variant and this is the one I am referring to. Methylfolate increases the production of these kinds of neurotransmitters and it can also help with the breakdown to some extent (through production of SAMe). In my experience, those with a homozygous COMT SNPs have a strong tendency toward restless sleep, difficulty falling asleep and anxiety. These symptoms are directly correlated with what the enzyme's function is. Because methylfolate can increase the production of these molecules that COMT helps to remove, those with co-occurring MTHFR often need less methylfolate (and they just don't seem to tolerate it) than their counterparts with normal (wild type) COMT function.

Instead, those with COMT often find taking magnesium to be as helpful, or more helpful, than methylfolate. This is because magnesium is one of the cofactors for COMT. SAMe is also a cofactor for COMT. While SAMe and methylfolate can be helpful, in my experience, much less of these are needed when both COMT and MTHFR (C677T) homozygous SNPs are present. When COMT homozygous is present, taking 200–400 mg of absorbable magnesium can go a long way to improving sleep, energy, mental function, and your tolerance to methylfolate.

MAOA (monoamine oxidase) and MAOB enzymes have a little overlap with COMT. These two enzymes are responsible for helping your body get rid of and detoxify serotonin, epinephrine, dopamine, histamine, and other amines. The MAOB is more specific to the stimulating neurotransmitters like epinephrine and dopamine. When there is a defect in this enzyme, the person may present similar to those with COMT SNPs. For instance, they may have increased anxiety, trouble with sleep, and irritability. Because of slowed histamine clearance they may also be more prone to angry outbursts. So, just like with COMT SNP, those with MAOA and MAOB will need to be more careful with their methylfolate dosing. The cofactor for this enzyme is riboflavin, which can help with the enzyme function and improve mood and tolerance for methylfoalte.

SOD or superoxide dismutase is the enzyme that helps your body eliminate or neutralize superoxide free radicals. These superoxide free radicals are a normal part of our biochemistry and are created during normal metabolism, fighting off microbes and other aspects of the immune system. However, when superoxide cannot be neutralized, it can lead to more problems from oxidative stress and inflammation. When you have mutations in the SOD gene, your super oxide dismutase enzyme will be slowed down, leading to more super oxide free radicals, increased inflammation and oxidative stress. This can lead to a slowing down in methylation enzyme function and other metabolic function. It can present in a lot of different ways but some symptoms include:

- Increased pain in muscles or joints
- More fatigue
- More headaches
- Weakness

As it relates to methylfolate higher doses of methylfolate could aggravate symptoms since it increases the cells' metabolic activity. As a result the cells will be producing more free radicals than you may be able to neutralize. This will lead to worsening or exacerbation of your symptoms.

Therefore, if you're introducing methylfolate into your system you need to be cautious when you have an SOD alteration, specifically SOD2 since it is in the mitochondria. If you have alterations in this enzyme you can take SOD in a capsule form away from food. Trace minerals are also helpful for this enzyme to function properly.

CBS is an enzyme that stands for cystathionine-beta-synthase and it is the first step in transforming sulfur molecules into other things like waste (ammonia urea, sulfites) and/or antioxidants like glutathione. It is not very common to have a lot of issues coming from CBS alone. When it does occur, it is part of a bigger picture, so let me explain in more detail.

CBS SNPs can either be up-regulated (sped up) or down-regulated (sped down). When someone has up regulation, they may need more support making glutathione and like need more vitamin B6 as this is the cofactor. In the cases of CBS up regulation, typically there is higher stress (higher cortisol) and high serum ammonia levels. This occurs because the up-regulated CBS enzyme sends more of your homocysteine into sulfur byproducts, which can lead to increased ammonia. Ammonia is a neuro-inflammatory molecule. As you might imagine, this inflammation in the nervous system can make one have anxiety and a lower pain threshold. These symptoms may wax and wane based on your ammonia levels.

So if you have an up regulation in your CBS (C699T) SNPs get your ammonia levels checked on several occasions to see if you are above 40 ng/dl. Keep in mind that not everyone with increased CBS will have higher ammonia; it will also depend on your other genetics and health factors.

As it related to methylfolate, a CBS up regulation should lead you to be more careful taking methylfolate. Methylfolate may lead to reduced levels of homocysteine leading to over-methylation. Oftentimes with CBS up regulation, homocysteine levels will be low. This is sign that you may have a CBS up regulation. I should also note that there are environmental factors that can also up-regulate your CBS enzyme, like infections and other sources of inflammation.

Increase

MTR, also known as methionine transferase, is the main enzyme that methylfolate and methylcobalamin are supporting. Genetic alterations in this (A2756G) enzyme usually result in a higher demand for these cofactors (methylfolate and methylcobalmin).

MTRR is a genetic alteration in the enzyme that recycles vitamin B12 so that your body can use it again. When this (A66G) SNP is present, your body will require higher amounts of B12 to function optimally. A daily dose is recommended and sometimes injections are needed. This is used in conjunction with methylfolate when needed but does not necessarily mean more methylfolate is needed. Because both support SAMe production, more may be needed depending on your MTHFR genetics and response to methylfolate.

Two other SNPs that change how much methylfolate you may need are GAMT and PEMT. These are both methyltransferase enzymes and require SAMe (as a cofactor) to do their job. Since methylfolate is needed to make SAMe and these enzymes need more SAMe to get adequate function, there is an increased demand for methylfolate. So when there are alterations in these enzymes (PEMT and GAMT), I generally suggest using more methylfolate. Sometimes it is easier and more effective if you just take what these enzymes make, phosphatidyle choline for PEMT and creatine for GAMT.

BHMT is also a methyltransferase enzyme. This enzyme has the ability to create SAMe without the use of methylfolate. The enzyme betaine-homocysteine methyltransferase combines homocysteine with betaine (aka trimethylglycine) to make SAMe. When there are alterations in the BHMT-02 and 08 versions, there seems to be more difficulty with focus and attention. I was not able to find any research to support this but have observed this in my practice (see the case study below for more specifics).

FOL corresponds to the folate receptor for absorbing folate into the body. The FOL-1 is responsible for absorbing methylfolate in particular. When a homozygous alteration is present here you may need to use a liposmal form of methylfolate.

Below, in the next section, we will discuss starting methylfolate, some mistakes I have made (in part 2) in treating people with MTHFR and some side effects and symptoms to be aware of when you begin.

Action Step

MTHFR is just one gene so consider having a broader SNP report generated from sources like strategene (from seekinghealth.com), mthfrdoctors.com geneticgenie.org, mthfrsupport.com and nutrahacker.com. Because these can be really complicated to look at and decide what is and is not important, consider consulting with a doctor who specializes in genetic medicine.

Step 5:
Titration and Dosing Adjustments

Your first dose of methylfolate should always be a small one since we want to make sure you don't have any side effects. Please note that Deplin does not come in a low dose. For those who are not familiar with it, Deplin is a prescription medical food that contains methylfolate. It is sold at pharmacies but only comes in doses of methylfolate of 7.5 and 15 mg. Because of the high dose, I would strongly discourage starting with this.

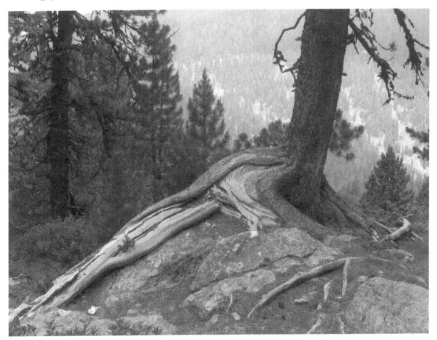

Adverse reactions are not typical when your body is low in methylfolate (positive for MTHFR mutation) but they can happen. They are more common when the "other genes" noted above are present. In this section we will discuss in more detail some of those reactions and what to do about them. By starting with the lowest dose for your particular MTHFR SNP (noted above) and working up, you should start to notice positive things like:

- Feeling more energetic
- Feeling in a better mood
- Feeling less brain fog
- Feeling less allergies
- Feeling less joint aches
- Feeling lighter in your body

Or on the negative side things like:

- Feeling worse
- Having headaches
- Having anxiety and trouble with sleep
- Feeling sluggish and heavy in your body
- Digestive problems like nausea, gas or bloating
- Rash or itchy skin
- More joint aches

Neither the negative nor the positive effects of methylfolate are going to happen with the first dose (typically). There is going to be a gradual change in how you feel over days, weeks or months.

Many times you will feel better at first but over time the adverse reactions will occur. This is especially true if you are pushing the upper limits of what your body can handle. The upper limit for you may not be the same as for someone else, so listen for these side effect sensations. When you have these, it is a sign that you need to reduce your dose, support other pathways, and look for other imbalances in the body. When you first start, I would even encourage you to reduce the dose if you have a day where you feel "great" or "better than you have in a while". This is the advice Dr. Ben Lynch encourages and I have found it to be true and accurate in my practice as well. You may think you have just the right dose and maybe you do, but the there is a thin line between just enough and too much. Those great feelings should be a signal that you are at the upper limit and you should be cautious about taking higher doses. It is easier to reduce the dose and feel not quite as good than to reverse the adverse reactions noted above (and below).

So if you are having a few really good days or weeks, try to reduce the dose a bit for one or two days and see how you feel. If you crash (all the old symptoms return), titrate the dose back up to where it was and stick with this dose moving forward. If you feel fine or better at the lower dose for 2–4 days you may want to take a few days off of your methylfoalte dosing per week. After you have been on the folate for several months you probably won't need to take days off at all. Since this is a bit tricky to figure out on your own, I recommend using some kind of physical tracking to reference over time. Below you will find a symptom tracker that was created just for this kind of tracking. You can use this tracker to help you and your doctor (if you are working with one) better understand the benefits (and potentially side effects) of taking methylfolate or other methylation support.

Anxiety/Stress/Irritability

When you have an MTHFR alteration, it may be the cause of some or all of your anxiety. However, we need to be cautious because methylfolate can also worsen or create anxiety too. When and if it happens, there are several reasons for this. The most common occurs when MTHFR treatment begins without taking into consideration the full effects of this treatment. For instance, with MTHFR treatment the idea is to correct for a deficiency (of methylfolate), but this can cause more problems when there are also deficiencies with other enzymes and pathways that methylfolate feeds into downstream.

What do I mean by downstream? Well, methylfolate is a key nutrient needed to make neurotransmitters. Increasing methylfolate in your body will typically result in more neurotransmitter production. However, if you have a genetic defect in the enzymes that break down neurotransmitters you will end up with an excess of neurotransmitters. This excess creates an anxious, irritable, and uncomfortable experience. Sometimes this reaction is severe, even bordering on psychosis, and at other times it creates a subtler irritability and anger. This phenomenon typically occurs when the person has COMT and MAOa and MAOb SNPs and at a dose of methylfolate above 4mg (it can also occur at much lower doses). When this occurs, the solution is to reduce the dose of methylfolate and look at the other biochemical pathways connected to methylfolate and methylation.

Ask yourself these two questions:

- Do you have a tendency toward anxiety already (more so than depression)?

- Do you have a tendency toward not sleeping well already?

- Do you have chronic allergies?

If you answered yes to any of these, you may be more susceptible to methylfolate side effects and worsening your sleep and anxiety. The question is how much is too much? Using the symptom tracker (below), you can track and find the right dose for you; however, if you want a deeper understanding of what is causing this reaction and what to do the sections below will provide more details. Many times (certainly not always) if you answer yes to the above questions you have some slowdown in neurotransmitter (amines including histamine) breakdown. Many times simply taking an absorbable form of magnesium will help speed up their breakdown and resolve these issues, even if a COMT SNP is not present.

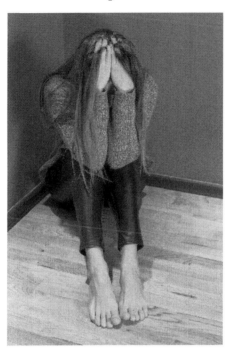

Joint Aches

Joint and body aches can occur from taking methylfolate and other methyl donors. Similar to the support of neurotransmitter production, methylfolate also supports the production of our cell membranes through helping produce SAMe. With the help of SAMe the enzyme PEMT then is able to produce cell membranes. Cell membranes are made up of fatty acids like phosphatidylcholine and other phospholipids. Production of these is needed regularly because there is always damage and repair occurring in our bodies.

For instance, each time we contract a muscle, small micro-tears occur in the muscles that perform the contraction. The cell membrane in these muscles then needs to be repaired. Methylfolate supports this process, that's the good part. However, if you take too much the whole process can be down-regulated or turned down by the body in a self-regulating effect.

In other words, when the body sees it has enough of a certain molecule (SAMe) it will down-regulate its production and the processes it is connected to. When that occurs, the person may experience aches in their joints and muscles from down regulation of cell membrane production. Once the levels of SAMe decrease, the process will restart again. I should note here that there are other reasons this can happen too (see digestive problems below).

If you do get joint aches and found that the methylfolate was helping the aches initially, consider taking phosphatidylcholine directly. This can be consumed in the form of a supplement in place of the methylfolate. It typically has fewer side effects than methylfoalte. The dose is about 1–2 grams per day. Use the symptom tracker to find the dose of either methylfolate or phosphatidylcholine where you feel best.

Digestive Problems

If you have made it this far you should have identified some digestive problems and tried to improve them or you did not think you had any digestive problems. If you have not done this, you should. Here is why. When we consume B vitamins and there are excess microbes in the small intestine, the microbes can and do eat them as well. When this happens, the B vitamins are turned into a different metabolite, which may not have a favorable effect on your body. This paper[8] explores this topic in detail and it is something I have seen clinically. Some people say, "I can't take B vitamins because they make me nauseous or cause abdominal pain." If this is you, there is likely a microbial overgrowth or imbalance problem.

Outside of microbial imbalance problems, poor digestion limits absorption of many micronutrients including folates, B vitamins, and many other minerals and micronutrients. If you think you have microbial imbalance you should try to sort through some of that before starting methylfolate. Two alternative routes are to take a liposomal form of methylfolate or use other methyl donors instead of methylfolate. This is discussed in more detail below.

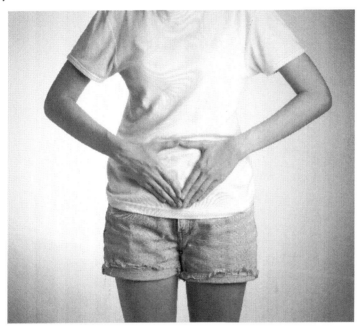

Headaches

MTHFR gene alteration can be a cause of headaches. However, headaches can be triggered when someone is being treated for MTHFR as well. Not everyone will experience them but in most cases they occur from taking too much (for you) folate or other methyl donors. The most common reason it happens is because the body has built-in negative feedback loops.

Just as with the cell membranes, when the body senses there are enough of certain substances, it shuts off production. This then shifts the flow of molecules into different pathways/directions. You could think of this similar to building a dam and using the water for irrigation. One switch will shift the water in a different direction. In the case of headaches, the switch pushes molecules (homocysteine) into a detoxification pathway. So the headaches come from the body increasing detoxification. Typically it is sulfur detoxification but could also be hormones and other molecules. At the same time you may experience bodily aches or a feeling of heaviness in the body as described above.

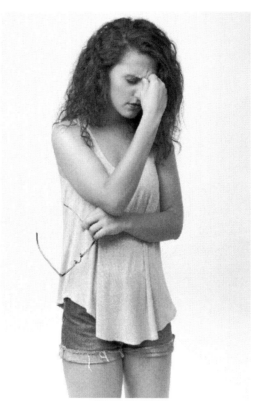

If this happens the main recommendation is to stop taking or reduce the methylfolate and support detoxification of sulfur and neurotransmitters with trace minerals and magnesium. Headaches can have multiple origins and may have nothing to do with taking methylfolate. In the case there is a clear connection, start by lowering the dose. If you feel good with a lower dose, you may not need to go higher and even worry about the headaches as an issue. In the case you are still not feeling well and think you need more methylation support, start adding some magnesium and trace minerals. Trace minerals are found in multivitamins but you can find them by themselves in the form of drops or capsules. Remember, if you use a multivitamin make sure it does not have folic acid in it. A pure trace mineral will be a more potent option. The case studies below discuss headaches in more detail.

Action Steps

If you are experiencing these side effects, consider taking a step back and evaluating your overall health especially your digestion, diet, and detoxification pathways.

If these are in good working order as far as you can tell, stop taking methylfolate and instead look at the cofactors for the SNPs listed above. For instance, you may need more magnesium for the COMT SNP or simply a trace mineral like molybdenum to support sulfur detoxification. Many people are magnesium and trace mineral deficient anyways. Trace minerals are required for almost every enzyme in our bodies to work properly and magnesium is needed to process many of the downstream metabolites of methylation.

Other options include taking methyl donors other than methylfolate as discussed in more detail below. Remember the symptom tracker below can be used to help guide you to clearly see how each addition or removal is affecting you. Use this carefully to see the patterns. If you cannot find the pattern you should do some testing to understand over-methylation or under-methylation. Two good options include serum homocysteine or SAMe/SAH ratio (speciality lab test) test.

Methylation Support Part 2

There are several other vitamins outside of methylfolate to consider for support of your overall methylation cycle. As with your need for methylfolate, your need for these vitamins and nutrients will be dependent on your other genetic alterations and other environmental influencers.

Let's say, for instance, that you don't know your other genetics but you determine you need several milligrams of methylfolate daily. After taking this for several weeks or months, you have not had any of the side effects noted above, you are feeling pretty good. This is great, but naturally with taking more methylfolate there is more methylation occurring. As a result, you need to support the other enzymes involved in methylation and enzymes downstream from methylation. This support would come in the form of the corresponding enzyme cofactors like B1, B2, B3, B6, B12, magnesium, and trace minerals. In some cases (based on your specific genetics and health issues) you may need these just as much or more than you need the methylfolate (depending on your genetics and environmental influencers). As a general rule, however, the more methylfolate you take the more cofactor support is needed to stay in balance. Once you get over 1000–2000mcg you will need to consider other cofactor support.

Vitamin B12 has a synergistic effect with methylfolate and should be taken in conjunction with methylfolate at minimum a few times per week and at maximum daily. If there are absorption issues and transportation issues (like the TCN2 SNP) in the genetics, sometimes injections of B12 are required. The standard dose for B12 is 1000mcg of methylcobalamin. To be safe, I always recommend taking it under the tongue or sublingually. This will have the best chance for absorption.

Trimethylglycine, or betaine, is another one that can provide additional support to methylation as does vitamin B6. Like the recommendations for methylfolate, it is difficult to give a general amount that everyone should take. One safe way to approach it is, as you are increasing your methylfoalte dose above 1–2 mg, start to add B-complex without folic acid. Take the B complex 1–2 times per week to start. Use the symptoms tracker when you make these changes so that you can clearly see how each addition or removal is affecting you. As you increase further you may need more targeted support.

Let's look at some real cases I have treated so you can get more context on what you should do in different situations. I specifically choose more challenging cases as this is always where the learning comes from.

Learning from My Mistakes: Case Studies

Two States, Tired and More Tired

The first woman came in wanting help with energy and depression. As she described it, "I have been fatigued and depressed my whole life." She also had immuno-deficiency syndrome. After failing multiple psychiatric medications, she got a genetic test done by her psychiatrist. This test revealed MTHFR (C677T homozygous) and she was put on Deplin and SAMe. As she reports it, "These did not help. I am still taking them, but they did nothing."

In addition to the fatigue and depression she had major headaches. The headaches were occurring every day. She also had numbness in her legs and chronic diarrhea. She had been screened by several gastroenterologists and did not have celiac disease (based on blood and biopsy), Crohn's or ulcerative colitis. She was diagnosed with IBS but not given any effective treatment.

The one thing that did work well for her was sleep. She never had any trouble sleeping her whole life. She slept about 9 hours per night but still felt very tired, rating her energy at 3–4/10. We did not have any other genetic information.

In the first visit, I asked her to stop the Deplin and SAMe as an experiment. She did this and reported that the headaches went away within a few days and were still gone. However, her depression and fatigue got worse. As part of the experiment I let her know if any of her symptoms got worse, she should restart the SAMe but not the Deplin. She did this and her mood improved but she was still depressed (no anxiety).

So what was triggering the headaches and what did we do to make them better? Why did her depression get worse rather than better? These are the questions we had to answer to take her case to the next level. The most obvious reason was over methylation because Deplin is very high dose methylfolate. However, she also had issues with digestion that cold be contributing.

Because she had chronic diarrhea and immunodeficiency, I was highly suspicious of a GI bug or bugs. The initial round of tests were negative. However, the low FODMAP diet seemed to improve her digestion as noted by a reduction in the amount of daily Imodium she needed to take. She was given a test for SIBO and in the meantime started taking phosphatidylcholine two pills twice daily.

She came back in four weeks and all of a sudden she could not fall asleep and was getting some anxious feelings. The sleep response was particularly interesting since she had previously stated she never had trouble falling asleep and slept 8–10 hrs. per day.

Since starting the phosphatidylcholine, her energy (rating it at 6–7/10) and mood were better. She was starting to get some headaches again but nothing like what she had initially. The results of her SIBO test were negative.

I asked her to decrease the phosphatidylcholine to just two per day and start taking magnesium at bedtime. She continued the low FODMAP diet. When she returned, she noted that the headaches had resolved and her sleep had improved. Her energy and mood were not quite as good, however.

We slowly added small amounts of methylfolate in a liposomal form for better GI absorption, about 100mcg per day. Any more than this and headaches would flare up along with poor sleep etc.

This case did take a few more turns and she is still actively being treated. At this point it seems whatever is going on with her digestion is holding back her progress. We are actively testing and treating this. The points I wanted to emphasize were her responses to the different methyl donors.

The first thing to note is that she was sensitive to methylfolate more so than SAMe and phosphatidylcholine. Her mood and energy do seem to respond to methyl donors but are easily pushed into over-methylation or increased detox and stimulation. I made the mistake of giving her too much methylation support without knowing how she would respond downstream.

I later found out that she does have a COMT (met/met). Since the phosphatidylcholine was preserving her methylfoalte she was able to make more neurotransmitters (serotonin, norepinephrine, dopamine). Since these are stimulating and keep people awake, she was not able to sleep because they are broken down in a large part by COMT. This explains at least some of the reason why she could not sleep when given higher amounts of methyl donors. Once this was identified and accounted for (with magnesium) she did much better. It is also worth noting that high dose of Deplin did not cause the same reaction as the phosphatidyle choline. This I slinky due to poor gi absorption of the Deplin. Overstimulation is the most common problem from methyl donors. Even if you feel tired now and think you always are tired and under stimulated, don't be surprised if this shifts in a dramatic way.

Sad and Sensitive

This case involves a person who self-reports being "sensitive" both emotionally and physically. Her main complaints are fatigue, depression, anxiety, and an uncomfortable feeling on her skin (mildly painful and sensitive to the touch but hard for her to explain), with some muscle pain. She does not sleep well and is always worried about side effects from medications and different products. She is the person who will inevitably get the side effects from a medication or nutrient if there is any possibility that they might occur.

At first, she seems like a good candidate for some methylation support but her sensitivity worried me initially. Perhaps her low energy and mood are from low folate and SAMe and her skin problems from underproduction of phosphatidyle choline.

After getting a more thorough understanding of her overall health, I learn that she recently started taking SAMe, L-tryptophan and L-tyrosine and feels better but she does not know which one of these three has helped her. She also mentions that she has some digestive problems, which she describes as "mild constipation." "This does not bother me much now since I avoid the foods that trigger it." We decide to do some lab and genetic testing to get a better understanding of where to start. I also recommended she stop the L-tyrosine and switch the L-tryptophan to 5-hydroxytryptophan.

She returns and notes that she is "about the same, maybe a little better." The labs come back showing a low normal homocysteine and low normal and RBC magnesium. The genetic tests are not back.

I recommend she take magnesium 400mg at bedtime, stop the SAMe and start phosphatidylcholine 800mg instead. She returns noting that her sleep and energy are a little better but she still is not sleeping great and her energy is still low (5/10). After reviewing her genetic SNPs we found that she has very mild MTHFR (one copy of 1298c) COMT (v178 heterozygous), PEMT (homozygous), MTRR (a66G heterozygous).

I recommended she increase her phosphatidylcholine to two per day and add methyl B12 1000 mcg per day, and increase the magnesium to 600–800 mg per day. She was limited on funds so we decided to see how this plan went for three months. She returned and said her energy was better (now rating at 6/10) and her sleep was too. She still had trouble sleeping at times and her skin sensitivity seemed to be a little worse, at least it was something that she talked about more.

I recommend she switch the phosphatidyle choline to phosphatidyle serine as this was more calming and she had a strong tendency toward anxiety anyway. For her skin I recommended she switch methyl b12 to hydroxy b12 and try that for a few weeks. I expected this would help her skin more if she had inflammation going on.

She returned reporting no change in the skin but that sleep was consistently good now. We did try a few more things for her skin, but nothing seemed to do much. What were we missing?

Was it true that "maybe this is just how I have to live," as she put it?

In hindsight it seems so obvious, but I was not sure what I was missing at the time. At some point she returned and the conversation steered back to her digestion. Still she mentioned that this, "does not bother me much." She was already gluten free and very careful with the foods she ate, having several food sensitivities. I suggested that she be tested for SIBO and it turned out that she had a major case of this. At present it appears that the bacterial overgrowth and the immune reaction to this are what are driving her skin sensitivity and likely some of the other health issues she has.

Tank on Empty

This is a 45-year-old male with some fatigue, mild exercise intolerance and occasional anxiety. His main concern was with exercise intolerance. After helping him improve his hormone levels this was better, but he still had some issues. The way he described it was, "I feel like I can't run past a certain point. I get to about 5 miles and just can't go any further or have to go really slow. It also seems like it takes longer for me to recover from exercise." He was interested in doing some longer endurance training but did not think he could do it because of these.factors

Overall his energy was at a solid 7/10 and he felt pretty good otherwise. After getting a broader understanding of his health it did not seem like there were any other obvious health issues. I thought he could be having some issues with methylation and it was driving his endurance and recovery issues. After all, methylation is needed for creatine production and cellular recovery. We looked at his serum homocysteine and it was 15 umol/L. So he decided he wanted to look at the genetic factors that could be driving this. What we found was that he had some alterations in two of his GAMT enzymes and had MTHFR (compound heterozygous) and MTRR (homozygous A66G).

I recommended he first start taking methylcobalmin (mb12)1000mcg and methylfolate 800mcg. Over the next two weeks we worked the methylfolate up to about 4 grams. After this add creatine 1500mg per day. He was also advised to avoid foods containing folic acid.

He returned 3 weeks later and reported no change, but after some conversation he admitted not taking the creatine at all and not being consistent in taking the other supplements. Sometimes he would forget to take them. To make it easier for him I told him, "If you do nothing else just take the creatine and even take higher doses when you are training."

I explained how the GAMT enzyme works and the importance of creatine in the body. GAMT is an enzyme that converts guanidinoacetate into creatine with the help of SAMe. His body was only doing this in a limited capacity. Creatine is one of the molecules that allow your body to keep going when you reach your anaerobic threshold. This was the exact reason he came in. He agreed to be more consistent and aggressive with the dosing and return in a month.

This time it worked; he was able to work out more frequently and at longer distances than ever before. His muscles were adapting to the training and with that so was his endurance.

Too Many Projects to Finish

Sometimes the simplest treatments are the most effective with lasting results. This next case illustrates this well. She was about 26 years old and came in accompanied by her mother. From what I could tell by body language she appeared to be in happy spirits. Upon digging deeper I discovered she was depressed and was having difficulty finding joy in the things that she used to enjoy.

Her depression would get really bad at times and she also had made a few suicide attempts. She did not know what triggered it. About eight months prior she was hospitalized after an attempt. She was given several antidepressant and antipsychotic medications, all of which seemed to worsen her depression and she stopped taking them. We did some labs and she returned in a few weeks.

The labs showed a high normal homocysteine, low protein, and a compound heterozygous MTHFR. Further conversation revealed that she was easily distracted and did not finish tasks that she stared. She did not have much anxiety and felt more down than anything. Her sleep was usually good.

ADD/ADHD symptoms such as difficulty finishing tasks and getting distracted easily are associated with under methylation. Trimethylglycine can be particularly helpful in the right person for these types of symptoms.

I asked her to increase her protein to about 1/2 her body weight in grams and start trimethylglycine (TMG) 750 mg per day in the a.m. She returned with improved energy and mood. She also stated that she had finished two projects that were on her to-do list for a long time.

It was hard for me to believe that such a simple thing could help so much. Her energy and mood were not perfect, but she was clearly better from what she and her mother said. While I was tempted to give her additional treatment and refinement, there was not much need. The only modification was to increase the TMG to two every other day.

When Everything Else Fails

When all your efforts are not working or you are just too confused about what to do next, start with this. You can call this the simple and easy way to treat MTHFR and methylation problems. It may not be as effective as the above mentioned but it is also better than nothing. In trying to narrow down methylation support to the simplest common denominators, partially for this book and partially for a clinical setting, I have distilled it down to main things:

1. Ensure optimal digestion and/or rule out any digestive problems.

2. Support collateral pathways, specifically COMT and histamine clearance.

Do these two things and you are more likely to experience the benefits of methylfolate and much less likely to have any of the methylfolate side effects discussed above. However, the degree to which you understand these two things will determine your ultimate success or failure with optimizing your methylation and folate status. I discussed digestive problems in some detail above. Sometimes people don't have digestive symptoms even though many of their health issues are coming from their digestive tract. If you keep running into problems with your treatment, I would recommend doing some advanced testing on your digestive tract like:

- Leaky gut - lactulose/mannitol or other intestinal barrier function assessment.

- Assessing your microbiome balance (or lack thereof)

- Rule out presence of pathogenic microbes using DNA detection methods rather than cultures.

I did discuss supporting collateral pathways above, but it is particularly important to support clearance of histamine, catecholamines, and other amines. The following vitamins and minerals are some of the cofactors that support the enzymes that allow for their clearance: magnesium, vitamin B6, vitamin B5, vitamin B1.

Note that methyl donors like methylcobalmin, methylfolate and SAMe are also needed for the clearance of histamine and other catecholamine. However, these will make things worse if the collateral pathways are not supported first. This is especially true for those that have genetic alterations in the enzymes responsible for amine clearance (COMT, MAOB, MAOA, HNMT, ABP1).

Step 6:
Navigating Nature vs. Nurture

"The first principal is that you must not fool yourself, and you are the easiest person to fool."

Richard Feynman

As I have alluded to throughout this book, the fate of your health is not solely tied to any one gene or your genetic code in general. The biochemical processes that stem from your genetics are an evolving dance between your genes and the environment. The ebb and flow of environmental triggers like infections, toxin exposure, and micronutrient deficiencies can shift your biochemistry ever so slightly or with robust vigor. The degree of impact each environment trigger has on your health is genetically determined. For instance, those with MTHFR may need longer to heal from cellular damage. So, for instance, if you get a cut on your skin or damage to your digestive tract it may take you longer to recover from that damage. This is because methylfolate is needed to repair those tissues. The same slowed recovery would occur in someone who has normal MTHFR genetics but is simply deficient in methylfolate.

Another environmental trigger that will shift your biochemistry is an infection. Most people can recover rapidly from acute infections, but months and years of chronic infections can cause some aspects of the body to be rundown. Some infections can specifically affect the methylation cycle leaving those with MTHFR even more rundown. These are just a few examples of how environmental triggers and genetics affect the biochemicals that ultimately impact your health.

With so many environmental variables and varying degrees of effects, I cannot give a one-size-fits-all treatment for your MTHFR defect. Instead, I suggest you start with the most common and obvious environmental triggers discussed in the epigenetic section. Do an honest self-assessment or go to your doctor and have them evaluate you for each of these. Remember, getting an opinion from an experienced clinician can be very useful as each of these can present in different ways.

I also discussed genetic variations, other than MTHFR, that will influence your biochemistry and the effect of your methylation treatment. All in all, the environmental triggers and genetic variables are the colors and shades that make up your health picture.

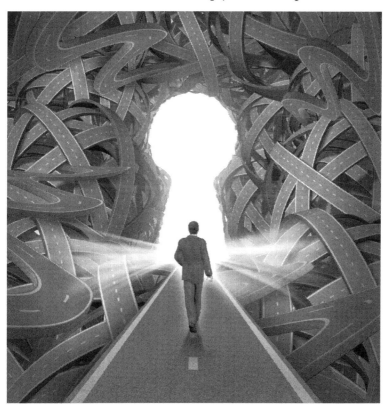

The information I presented here are just models to guide you to more predictable (and hopefully desired) results. Remember, though, the model is not the actual. Your body is the actual. Only you have direct access to your feelings, emotions, and symptoms. Use these models as a starting point but make them your own. If you are not getting the results you expect, it suggests something in the model is not right and may need to be adjusted. If you follow this approach, you will continually refine a clearer and clearer picture of your health. The clearer the picture of the problem the more open the path toward better health.

With this in mind, I always recommend my patients track their symptoms and try to find the things that influence or are associated with their symptoms. This can be very helpful in finding the underlying cause you and your doctor are searching for. That is not to say that everything you associate with your symptoms will be related to the underlying cause, but it can be very helpful in finding out what the cause is.

What follows are a few questions to continually refine your model as you explore your health through optimizing methylation. Ask yourself these questions once weekly when you first start and regularly after that until you are satisfied with all the aspects of your health picture. These are some of the questions I would be asking you if you were coming into my office for face-to-face visits. Following the questions is the "Symptom Tracker." Use this to track your progress and structure the changes you make to your health regimens like starting methylfolate, increasing the dose, changing your diet or other changes.

Remember health is not static. With any change you make (diet, supplement or other) be on the lookout for changes in your health, your symptoms and signs (like labs), and how you feel generally. Don't wait until things are really bad to try to locate the source or seek outside help.

General questions to explore environmental impact on your health

- What foods do you feel best with? Why?
- Is there a way to look at the foods that impact you as a category?
- How do you respond in different environments? Why do you think that is?
- Do certain seasons or weather patterns seem to bring on health ailments? Why?
- How do you feel at work versus home?
- How does stress affect your symptoms?
- Is there anything different about your symptoms when you are on vacation that suggests your home is causing your symptoms?

Questions after starting methylfolate

- Since starting the methylfolate do you feel better, worse or the same?
- Have you had any headaches or have your headaches increased?
- Do you feel more anxious and worried or excited and free?
- Does your body have a heavy feeling?

Most of the answers to these questions were covered in the book and should be fairly obvious. An experienced doctor can give you a lot of insight with just a few questions and help you find the reason why you are not getting better or are struggling to see the full picture. This book is not intended to replace clinical insight from a doctor but to give you the framework to ask the right questions both of yourself and your doctor.

The Symptom Tracker

Using the Tracker

What symptom or symptoms are you trying to improve? Start by picturing or feeling that symptom in your mind's eye. Once you have a good picture in your mind's eye, try to name the symptoms or cluster of problems you are trying to improve. It does not have to be a known symptom or problem. In fact, it is probably better if you describe it in your own terms, whatever words you think capture the essence or feeling of the problem, but it doesn't have to be perfect either.

Next, using the symptom rater, rate the severity of your symptom. Here I would encourage using the positive aspect of the symptom. This is what I mean; if you have fatigue (low energy), you want to rate your energy rather than your fatigue. Since more energy is what you want, we want to track it as this improves over time. If you have some annoying skin sensitivity, you would be rating the presence of normal skin sensation. Normal skin sensation would be a 5 and really abnormal would be a 1.

Intervention

Now, what substance or diet change are you going to use to see if you can have an effect on this symptom(s)? Write this in the line provided. It is recommended that you choose one or the other. For instance, don't do a diet and a supplement at the same time until you know how each is going to impact the symptom separately.

Next, in the table, write today's date and your rating of your symptom as a starting place. In the line below write the date range you will be taking the substance or diet change. The date range should correspond to how long you expect to be taking the substance to actually start to see a change. It might be a good idea to do a little research; try to find out how long the diet or supplement might take to have an effect. It does not have to be certain. Writing it down, though, will keep you honest about when to move on to something else. A few days to a few months is the time range you should be thinking about. If it is a long period you may want to break it up and track 1–2 weeks separately. If the dose will change from one week to the next you should also track these dosages separately. Use one sheet for each symptom you have and each substance or diet you do. At the end of the date range you will rate your symptom again and place it in the symptom rating box.

The "adverse/unexpected" section is to document any unusual feeling or symptoms that come up (during the date range you are taking this substance and dosage) as well as things that seem like an adverse reaction. If you change your diet and you feel hungry all the time or thirsty, these will all be examples of things to keep track of so you can reference them later.

The "other influencing factors" is a place to note any behaviors, environmental things or activities that could have positively or negatively skewed the results; for instance, if you were traveling and did not get good sleep or you were on vacation and were able to sleep in more. Both of these might have a corresponding negative or positive impact on your energy or mood. You do not want to falsely attribute these to the diet change or substance you are taking. So it is a good idea to think back on things that may have occurred during this date range.

Potential side effects should be researched and listed for quick reference prior to starting. There may not be any but it is a good idea to know ahead of time. Expected outcome should be listed ahead of time as well. Again, the whole point of tracking is to avoid self-deception. What do you hope will improve from taking this substance or diet change? One small way to put it would be to increase energy from 2 up to 3 (or 5). After the date range you can go back and look to see what impact there was.

This is referred to as a treatment trial. Writing these details down as opposed to keeping them in your head and guessing is worth the small effort in the long run. If you are tracking this over six months are you really going to remember all these details like you do as you progress along? For most people it is highly unlikely.

Case Example

This case example is based on the case above, "Tank on Empty." Walking through this case with the tracker will give you a better understanding of how to effectively use the tracker.

This case was a 45-year-old male with some fatigue, mild exercise intolerance, and occasional anxiety. His main concern was with exercise intolerance. I won't reiterate the whole case here, but see how his case looks on the tracker below.

One last thing to consider; remember that just because certain things seem to be correlated and related does not always mean that they have a causal relationship. For instance, the rates of violent crimes and murder seem to rise in a similar pattern as ice cream sales do. However, we would not conclude that ice cream is causing violent crimes and murder. The same can be said for other associations you find. You may be tempted to assume a causal relationship. By confirming the assumption you will be less likely to be fooled, but be sure to stay diligent and open to other possibilities even when it seems like you have found a causal relationship. Being open-minded to finding more relationships and understanding how your body works is just as important as finding them.

Symptom Tracker (Example)

Symptom(s):_____Energy/Endurance_____

Substance(s):_____MB12__and 800mcg mfolate

Specific Diet:___avoid folic acid_____

Date	Symptom Rating	Dosage / Frequency	Adverse / Unexpected	Other Influencing Factors
Start 10/18/18	2.0			
10/18/17– 11/01/17	2.0	1000mcg SL Mb12/d+ 800 mfolate 2x/d	None	increased greens in diet
11/02/17– 11/16/17	2.0	1000mcg SL Mb12/d+ 1600 mfolate 2x/d		increased greens in diet
11/22/17– 12/13/17	4	Krealkaline 1.5 grams/d	None	increased greens in diet

Potential Side Effects: anxiety, poor sleep, heart palpitations

Expected Outcome: more endurance, energy, and better mood

Additional Comments: None

Blank Sample Pages

Symptom Organizer

Specific	Non-Specific	Other

Symptom Tracker

Symptom(s):_____

Substance(s)_____

Specific Diet_____

Symptom Rater				
1	2	3	4	5

Date	Symptom Rating	Dosage / Frequency	Adverse / Unexpected	Other Influencing Factors

Potential Side Effects:

Expected Outcome:

Additional Comments:

Author Bio

Doctor Terranella has been practicing integrative medicine for over 10 years in Phoenix, Arizona. During this time, he has helped hundreds of patients uncover the underlying cause(s) of their health issues. He often finds that genetics and digestion are at the heart of chronic health issues. Because our digestion feeds the rest of our bodies with nutrients, he believes it to be one of the core foundations of health. In fact, digestive problems are often the cause of chronic health issues.

The expression of poor genetics prevents chronic health issues from getting better in a timely manner. Many people don't realize how malleable their bodies are despite their genetics. Understanding your genetics empowers you with more context to understand why your health issues are manifesting the way they are. By using knowledge of both digestion and genetics more people can gain a deep understanding of what is causing their health issues. That's why he felt compelled to share this information with the world.

Doctor Terranella attended medical school at Bastyr University and received a doctorate in naturopathic medicine in 2006. He also received a degree in acupuncture from Wu Hsing Tao. He has been practicing integrative medicine since 2007 through which he helps many patients achieve and understand better health. Currently he is practicing at Southwest Integrative Medicine (swintegrativemedince.com).

I hope you enjoyed the book! If you did please leave a review on amazon. If you have questions about the content or other questions or concerns please send me an email drt@swintegrativemedicine.com and I would be happy to help.

References

[1] https://www.ncbi.nlm.nih.gov/books/NBK3794/

[2] http://mthfr.net/mthfr-mutations-and-the-conditions-they-cause/2011/09/07/

[3] https://www.healio.com/psychiatry/journals/psycann/2014-4-44-4/%7B3997d915-c68f-427d-a31d-68aa2593576b%7D/the-role-and-postulated-biochemical-mechanism-of-l-methylfolate-augmentation-in-major-depression-a-case-report

[4] https://discover-holistic-health-academy.thinkific.com/courses/digestive-apprentice

[5] https://www.ncbi.nlm.nih.gov/pubmed/22810216

[6] http://ewg.org/

[7] http://primarypsychiatry.com/wp-content/uploads/import/Pamlabs6big.jpg

[8] https://genomemedicine.biomedcentral.com/articles/10.1186/s13073-016-0296-x

Printed in Poland
by Amazon Fulfillment
Poland Sp. z o.o., Wrocław

89035886R00049